THE OBAMA HEALTH LAW: DANGEROUS TO YOUR HEALTH AND FREEDOM

THE OBAMA HEALTH LAW is a bruising blow to American freedom and medical excellence. But the war is not over. It cannot be. There can be no negotiation between freedom and coercion.

The White House has launched a 50-state public relations campaign to convince the public that the law enacted against their will is to their benefit. We cannot falter now. With the U.S. Constitution on our side and the hearts and minds of the American people with us, freedom will prevail. Please use the information contained in this Broadside to alert your fellow patriots to the dangers of this new law. It will lower your standard of care, put the government in charge of your care, and take away something as precious as life itself: your liberty.

There are better ways to improve health

[

insurance and help the uninsured. Congress should rip up the 2,700-page Obama health legislation and enact a 20-page law in plain, honest English – a law that members of Congress can actually read before voting on it.

Will the New Obama Health Law Affect Me?

Yes. The law requires almost everyone to enroll in a one-size-fits-all "qualified" health plan, beginning in 2014. When you file your taxes, you must attach proof that you are enrolled. The law gives the IRS new powers to track you down and penalize you if you don't comply.

The law also empowers the Secretary of Health and Human Services to make the important decisions: what "qualified" plans cover, how much you will be legally required to pay, and how much leeway your doctor will have.

The Obama health law also transfers decision-making power from your doctor to the federal government. Even if you are insured by Aetna, Cigna, or another private company and pay the premium yourself, the govern-

SEC. 1311(h)(1). *Beginning on January 1, 2015, a qualified health plan may contract with —*

(B) a health care provider only if such provider implements such mechanisms to improve health care quality as the Secretary may by regulation require.

ment is still in charge. You are required to be in a "qualified" plan, and qualified plans can pay only doctors who implement whatever regulations the Secretary of Health and Human Services imposes in the name of improving health care "quality." That covers everything in medicine – whether a doctor should use a stent or do a bypass surgery, or when to perform a cesarean section.

Under the new law, physicians are required to enter their patients' treatments into an electronic database, and that data will be monitored by the government. Doctors will be instructed on what the government deems to be cost-effective and appropriate care. The result is that doctors will be forced to choose between doing what their patient needs and avoiding a government penalty.

This is a huge loss of medical privacy and freedom. Never before has the federal government dictated how doctors treat privately insured patients, except on narrow issues such as drug safety. The Constitution does not permit it.

Welfare Reform in Reverse

The new health law creates $917 billion in entitlements through 2019 and possibly twice that cost in the second decade. It loosens the eligibility rules for Medicaid and adds 18 million people to the rolls, nearly doubling Medicaid enrollment. The law also creates a brand-new entitlement for moderate-income households (earning up to $88,000 a year) to get taxpayer-funded subsidies for private insurance.

Half of the price tag for these new entitlements is paid for with tax hikes, but the other half comes from slashing future funding for Medicare by $575 billion through 2019. People who have paid into the system their whole working lives and are counting on it will get less care, because the money is being shifted to support a vast expansion of government dependents.

TREATING SENIORS LIKE CLUNKERS

Everyone knows that if you don't pay to maintain and repair your car, you limit its life. The same is true as human beings age. We need medical care to avoid becoming clunkers – disabled, worn out, and parked in nursing homes and wheelchairs. For nearly half a century, Medicare has enabled seniors to get that care.

The Obama health law reduces future funding for Medicare by $575 billion over the next decade, just when 30 percent more people will be entering Medicare as the baby boomers turn 65. Those numbers don't add up. Baby boomers who are counting on Medicare will get less care than seniors currently get.

Most of the Medicare cuts are made by slashing what hospitals, home care services, and other institutions are paid to care for elderly patients. Cuts are even made to hospice care and dialysis care, opening an express lane to the cemetery. Defenders claim the Medicare cuts will eliminate fraud and abuse, not care. If this were true, wouldn't the government have eliminated the fraud and abuse already? In truth, only 1 percent of the cuts will come from fraud and abuse, the Congressional Budget Office estimates.

RICHARD FOSTER, chief actuary for the Centers for Medicare & Medicaid Services:

Thus, providers for whom Medicare constitutes a substantive portion of their business could find it difficult to remain profitable and, absent legislative intervention, might end their participation in the program (possibly jeopardizing access to care for beneficiaries).

"Estimated Financial Effects of the 'Patient Protection and Affordable Care Act,' as Amended," CMS, April 22, 2010, 10.

Slashing Medicare payments will force institutions to cut back on care for seniors. Richard Foster, chief actuary for the Centers for Medicare & Medicaid Services, warns that cuts will be severe enough to force 15 percent of institutions into the red, and some hospitals may have to stop accepting Medicare. Where will seniors go when their local hospital no longer takes Medicare?

In the past 40 years, hip and knee replacements, bypass surgeries, angioplasties, and cataract operations have transformed the experience of aging. Older people used to be trapped in wheelchairs with crippling arthritis or stuck in nursing homes with clogged arteries. But these procedures have significantly reduced disability among the elderly, as a September/October 2007 *Health Affairs* study shows. Elderly people are more active – volunteering, shopping, and enjoying their grandchildren. The Obama health law will undo this progress by reducing access to care.

The new law also expressly authorizes the Secretary of Health and Human Services to modify or eliminate preventive services for seniors based on the recommendations of the U.S. Preventive Services Task Force, the group that recently raised public outrage by saying women ages 40–49 and older than 74 should no longer get routine annual mammograms. A half-page later, the law empowers the secretary to increase preventive services for Medicaid recipients. The agenda couldn't be clearer.

Beware of more Medicare funding cuts to come. The law establishes an Independent Medicare Advisory Commission to make further reductions while shielding members of Congress from public outrage.

Driving this evisceration of Medicare are dangerous misconceptions, misuses of scientific data, and a dismissal of older people as not worth the upkeep.

Less Care Is Not *the Answer*

President Obama and his budget director, Peter Orszag, have told seniors not to worry about the funding cuts, claiming that Medicare spending could be cut by as much as 30 percent without doing harm. They cite the *Dartmouth Atlas of Health Care 2008*, which tries to prove that patients who get less care – fewer hospital days, doctor's visits, and imaging tests – have the same medical "outcomes" as patients who get more care. But read the fine print.

The Dartmouth authors arrived at their dubious conclusion by restricting their study to patients who died. They examined what Medicare paid to care for these chronically ill patients in their last two years. By definition, the outcomes were all the same: death. The Dartmouth study didn't consider patients who recovered, left the hospital, and even resumed active lives. It would be important to know whether these patients survived because they received more care.

The journal *Circulation* addresses that question in its Oct. 20, 2009, issue and disputes the Dartmouth conclusion. Examining patients with heart failure at six California teaching hospitals, doctors found that hospitals giving

SEC. 4105(a). EVIDENCE-BASED COVERAGE OF PREVENTIVE SERVICES IN MEDICARE.

(n) AUTHORITY TO MODIFY OR ELIMINATE COVERAGE OF CERTAIN PREVENTIVE SERVICES. — Notwithstanding any other provision of this title, effective beginning on January 1, 2010, if the Secretary determines appropriate, the Secretary may –

(1) modify –

(A) the coverage of any preventive service described in subparagraph (A) of section 1861(ddd)(3) to the extent that such modification is consistent with the recommendations of the United States Preventive Services Task Force. . . .

more care saved more lives. In hospitals that spent less, patients had a smaller chance of survival. That's the opposite of what Obama claims.

* * *

Most Doctors Do Not Knowingly Waste Money on Dying Patients

Newsweek's cover story on Sept. 21, 2009, "The Case for Killing Granny," published at the height of the debate over the Obama health care bill, argued that "the need to spend less money on the elderly at the end of life is the elephant in the room in the health-reform debate." Politicians pressing for "reform" frequently implied that money was being poured into treatments for dying patients who would not benefit.

Numerous studies prove that this is generally false. In 2006, Emory University researchers examining the records of patients in the year before they died found that doctors spend far less on patients who are expected to die than on patients expected to survive.

The Emory researchers said it's *untrue* that "lifesaving measures for patients visibly near death account for a disproportionate share of spending." They also found that doctors often can't predict when a patient is in the last year of life. The most expensive patients are those who showed every sign of being able to recover and then didn't.

In any case, the Obama health law's across-the-board reductions in funding for Medicare won't simply reduce end-of-life care; they will also reduce care for patients who are perfectly capable of surviving their illnesses and going on with life.

Increasing Longevity Is Not Bankrupting Medicare

Access to medical breakthroughs has resulted in huge improvements in longevity and quality of life. Life expectancy at age 65 has jumped from 79 years to 84. The harshest misconception is that this improvement in life expectancy is a burden on society. Wrong. Medicare data show that a patient who dies at 67 spends three times as much on health care at the end of life as a patient who lives to 90. Medicare data also prove that after age 70, patients tend to spend the same amount cumulatively on medical care whether they live another five years or another 25 years. Patients who live longer tend to spend far less per year and much less at the end of life.

What is costly is when seniors become disabled. Fortunately, access to care is not only lengthening life but also reducing disability. And nondisabled seniors use only one-seventh as much health care as disabled seniors. As a result, the annual increase in per capita health spending on the elderly is less than on the rest of the population.

It's true that Medicare is running out of money, but the medical breakthroughs that are enabling people to live longer are not the problem. There are too many seniors compared to the number of workers supporting the system with payroll taxes. This temporary imbalance is due to the post-World War II baby boom. To remedy the problem, the Congressional Budget Office has suggested inching up the eligibility age by one month per year (with an almost imperceptible impact on people nearing retirement) or asking wealthy seniors to pay more. These are reasonable solutions; reducing access to treatments is not. Medicare has made living to a ripe old age a good value. ObamaCare will undo that.

The cuts in future Medicare funding – which Obama calls "savings" – will mean less help in coping with aging and possibly shorter lives. Do we as a nation really want to treat seniors like clunkers?

Ripping up Your Constitutional Rights

The Obama health law robs you of your constitutional rights. Several provisions fail the constitutionality test and reveal Congress's disrespect for the public and the rule of law. To halt this attack on your liberty, we must advance to the next battlegrounds – the U.S. courts and the voting booth.

Making Health Insurance Compulsory

States are in revolt against the requirement that nearly every person enroll in a "qualified health plan." Numerous state governments

(21 as this Broadside goes to press) are filing lawsuits challenging mandatory health insurance. Forcing people to buy it obviously reduces the number of uninsured. But Congress doesn't have the authority to force people to buy a product.

Sen. Orrin Hatch (R-Utah) agrees. Before the law was enacted, he cautioned his Senate colleagues, "[I]f Congress may require that individuals purchase a particular good or service ... [w]e could simply require that Americans buy certain cars.... For that matter, we could attack the obesity problem by requiring Americans to buy fruits and vegetables."

Some members of Congress claim the "general welfare clause" of the Constitution empowers them to impose an insurance mandate. But they're taking the phrase out of context. The Constitution gives Congress power to tax and spend consistent with the general welfare, not to make other kinds of laws solely because they are for the general welfare.

The Obama health law expressly claims

that the interstate commerce clause of the Constitution gives Congress the authority to force everyone to buy insurance. But for half a century, states have regulated health insurance. In fact, individuals are barred from buying a health plan in any state except where they live, the antithesis of interstate commerce.

In the past, congressional majorities frequently resorted to the commerce clause to try justifying expansive lawmaking. They did not always succeed. In President Roosevelt's first term, Congress enacted the National Industrial Recovery Act (NIRA), claiming power to micromanage local businesses, set wages and hours, and even regulate how customers selected live chickens at the butcher. Four Brooklyn brothers, owners of Schechter Poultry Corp., a kosher chicken market, challenged the NIRA. The Schechters said Congress had no authority to interfere with their local business – that there was nothing interstate about it. The brothers took their case all the way to the U.S. Supreme Court and won. Their victory proves that in extraordinary times, it takes ordinary people to stand up for freedom.

Since the Schechter decision, the Supreme Court has stretched the meaning of interstate commerce to allow Congress to intrude in many areas. Yet in 1995, the high Court struck down a federal ban on guns in school zones, admonishing Congress that its power under the commerce clause still has limits, no matter how good the intentions. Congress was told to leave it to the states to police school zones.

Ten years later, congressional health "reformers" hoped that the U.S. Supreme Court's 2005 decision in *Gonzales v. Raich*, defining "interstate commerce" very broadly, would give them a constitutional EZ Pass to enact national health care. In that 2005 case, the Supreme Court ruled that the federal government could stop Angel Raich from consuming homegrown marijuana for medical purposes, even though it was permitted in her state and advised by her doctor. Amazingly, the Court said her homegrown supply – six stalks in all – amounted to interstate commerce because it could have a "substantial effect on supply and demand in the national market for that commodity."

In September 2005, Sen. Patrick Leahy (D-Vt.) grilled John Roberts, then the nominee for chief justice, demanding assurances that he would stand by the *Raich* ruling instead of trying to restrain congressional lawmaking on health care. The surprise came in the Supreme Court's next term, when in the words of Justice Clarence Thomas, the Court made a "hasty retreat" from *Raich*. In *Gonzales v. Oregon* in 2006, the Court left the issue of federal intervention in medical issues unanswered.

This is the setting for the states currently suing to challenge compulsory insurance. Although the smart money is usually on the Court upholding an act of Congress, Congress's claim that *not* purchasing a product (health insurance) affects interstate commerce may be too implausible for the justices to accept.

* * *

Medical Autonomy and Privacy

As important as these state challenges to compulsory insurance are, they gloss over an issue that is more consequential to our health and longevity: Can the federal government dictate how doctors treat their patients?

During the past half-century, the Supreme Court has established a zone of privacy protected by the Constitution. It includes a couple's choice to use contraception recommended by their physician (*Griswold v. Connecticut*, 1965) and a woman's choice to have an abortion provided by her physician (*Roe v. Wade*, 1973). How can freedom to make these choices with your doctor be protected, but not freedom to choose a hip replacement or a cesarean section? Either your body is protected from government interference or it's not.

The Obama health law requires that nearly everyone enroll in a "qualified" plan, then it says plans can pay only doctors who implement whatever regulations the Secretary of Health and Human Services imposes to improve health care "quality" (Section 1311). That covers everything in medicine. If challenged, this provision is likely to meet disapproval from a pro-privacy Court.

Consider how the high Court ruled one year after the *Raich* decision. Oregon had passed a Death with Dignity Act that set standards for doctors to administer lethal drugs to terminally ill patients who request them. The Bush administration argued that assisted suicide was not "legitimate" medical care; therefore, federal agents could halt the use of the drugs.

The Supreme Court ruled 6–3 against the Bush administration's interference in *Gonzales v. Oregon* (2006). Such intrusion, the Court said, "would effect a radical shift of authority from the States to the Federal Government to define general standards of medical practice in every locality." That's what the Obama health law does.

For example, it requires doctors to record patients' treatments in an electronic medical database and monitors doctors' decisions. Dr. David Blumenthal, the Obama administration's national coordinator for health information technology, explained in *The New England Journal of Medicine* in April 2009 that "embedded clinical decision supports" – his euphemism for computers telling doctors what to do – will manage the quality of doctors' decisions. The Supreme Court is likely to view these controls as a "radical shift" in authority from the states to the federal government, and even more importantly, a threat to privacy rights.

Before the current health care debate, the public discussed government interference in medical decisions largely in one context: abortion. When a lower federal court struck down the Partial-Birth Abortion Ban Act in 2004 (a decision later reversed by the Supreme Court), Planned Parenthood President Gloria Feldt said, "This ruling is a critical step toward ensuring that women and doctors – not politicians – can make private, personal health care decisions." During the litigation, federal authorities requested access to medical records to determine whether the partial-birth procedure was ever medically necessary. Privacy advocates defeated nearly every request.

Advocates for women's rights need to reassess the impact of the new health law. Whether you are a man or a woman, pro-choice or pro-life, you lose freedom and privacy under this law.

Violating the Takings Clause

The "takings clause" of the Fifth Amendment bars the government from taking your property without compensation. It should protect everyone, no matter how unpopular – even insurance companies – but Congress ignored it in writing the health bill. The Senate version goes beyond reining in insurance company abuses, a just cause, and actually caps insurance company profit margins at well below current levels, robbing shareholders.

Next year, Congress could impose similar caps on profit margins of bodegas, pizzerias, and grocers by arguing that food – also a necessity – is too expensive. Your business could be next.

In 2010, ordinary citizens will have to stand up for their constitutional rights, just as the Schechter brothers did 75 years ago. Members of Congress swear to uphold the Constitution, but it appears many are ignorant of what it says.

Deficit Reduction Is a Shell Game

The president's Bipartisan Commission on Fiscal Responsibility and Reform plans to take American taxpayers to the cleaners. The new commission is charged with reducing the gap between what the federal government spends and what it takes from taxpayers.

It met for the first time April 27, 2010, 35 days after the president signed his health law creating $917 billion in new entitlements through 2019 and possibly twice that cost in the second decade. These entitlements include doubling the size of Medicaid at a cost of $410 billion through 2019 and promising households earning up to $88,000 a year taxpayer-funded subsidies for private health plans.

Now, with the ink barely dry on the health

law, the big spenders call for fiscal responsibility. If your spouse went on a spending binge, came home laden with shopping bags, then announced that it was time for the family to go on a budget, what would you do? You'd insist that the latest purchases go back before the rest of the family is made to sacrifice anything.

Step one toward fiscal responsibility is repealing the Obama health law. Americans don't have to tolerate unfair insurance practices. Barring these practices takes up about 24 pages of the 2,700-page health law. These reforms can be enacted separately. Repealing the health law would mean sending back the big-ticket items – those brand-new entitlements with the price tags still on them – before they go into effect in 2014.

Amazingly, the president crisscrossed the country claiming that the new health law is "paid for" and "reduces the deficit." He omitted to say that it was paid for by raising taxes by $500 billion *and* eviscerating Medicare.

Expanding federal programs and paying for them with a half-trillion dollars in new taxes is not deficit reduction. It is freedom reduction.

When commission member Rep. Paul Ryan of Wisconsin said the focus should be on reining in government spending, Rep. Steny Hoyer, (D-Md.), majority leader of the U.S. House of Representatives, wrote in *The Wall Street Journal* on April 28, 2010, that the commission should take a more "balanced approach that shares the burdens fairly," meaning raising taxes.

Hoyer treated reducing spending and increasing taxes as morally equivalent options. They are not. Raising taxes reduces individual liberty.

The national sales tax already being discussed – a VAT – would affect everyone. In Europe, VAT stands for "value-added tax," a sales tax collected at each stage of a product's production and distribution. Although the phrase "value added" has a positive connotation, there is nothing positive about it. In the U.S., a VAT should be called a Vanishing America Tax, because it would erode our freedom and standard of living.

In many European countries, VATs started small but now add as much as 25 percent to the cost of an item, such as a car. The tax is hidden in the price – not added at the cash register – so when the government raises taxes to satisfy new demands for revenue, few shoppers realize tax increases are to blame for higher prices. VATs have diminished the purchasing power of European families and would do the same to American families.

Despite the president's repeated pledge not to raise taxes except on the rich, he says now that all options will be considered. Commission Co-Chairman Erskine Bowles announced on April 27, 2010, that the president says "he will support the conclusions of this committee, if we have the courage to make the recommendations."

Those recommendations will be announced Dec. 1, 2010, after the midterm congressional elections. The timing is sheer trickery. Recommendations should be announced well in advance of the election, giving voters time to grill congressional candidates on where they stand. The timing deprives the public of input – in effect, taxation without representation.

The timing is wrong, and so is the mission – deficit reduction. What the country needs is a spending reduction commission with experts largely from the private sector. The president's commission is dominated by former and current government officials. Most of these commissioners are addicts – hooked on spending taxpayers' money.

In contrast, a spending reduction commission drawn from outside Washington, D.C., would immediately see the moral imperative to repeal the Obama health law.

Even before the health law was enacted, the government was growing beyond the consent of the governed. In fiscal year 2009, local, state, and federal governments together spent 40 percent of everything produced in the U.S. In many European countries, government spending consumes half or more of everything produced to support government-run health care and government intrusions into many other aspects of life. When the government spends so much, less is left for people to spend as they choose.

Only once before in American history did government spending cross the 40 percent line – to wage World War II. Nothing today justifies a similar confiscation of nearly half of people's resources.

Amazingly, although the 40 percent mark was crossed, Congress plowed ahead and enacted the huge health care entitlements, claiming they were fine because of the tax hikes. That makes it clear that the *cause célèbre* in Washington – deficit reduction – is a shell game. In plain English, it means raising your taxes to keep pace with government spending.

Members of Congress need to be reminded that government spending should not consume 40 percent of all we are capable of producing. If they can't remember that number, they should write it on their palms. Americans don't want to be Europeanized.

* * *

Advocates for overhauling American medicine try to bamboozle the public into believing that other countries offer better care at a lower cost. On *Meet the Press* in August 2009, Tom Daschle, designated by President Obama to be his Secretary of Health and Human Services, said that Americans were spending too much and getting poor quality care. "The World Health Organization listed us 37th, just below Costa Rica and above Slovenia," said Daschle, arguing for an immediate overhaul. Daschle was referring to a report issued in 2000 by the World Health Organization.

That WHO ranking – 37 – became a compelling statistic in the national debate. It was cited on NPR's *Morning Edition* on Aug. 18, 2009. A *St. Louis Post Dispatch* editorial on Sept. 4, 2009, cited it as proof that action was needed. The *St. Petersburg Times* used it to rebut Sen. John McCain's claim the U.S. has the best health care in the world.

Then, on April 22, 2010, just a month after Obama's law was signed, the truth came out about the number 37. Dr. Philip Musgrove, editor in chief of the WHO Report 2000, announced in *The New England Journal of Medicine* that it was "long past time for this zombie number to disappear from circulation." He called the ranking "meaningless." "This is not simply a problem of incomplete, inaccurate, or noncomparable data; there are also sound reasons to mistrust the conceptual framework behind the estimates...."

Well said, Dr. Cosgrove, although a bit tardy. The WHO deemed the U.S. No. 1 for "responsiveness to the needs of patients." But the U.S. was demoted to 37th for "overall performance," because the WHO report gave far more credit overall to countries where government finances all health care, calling it fairer than a market system.

Also influential was a bag-of-tricks report from The Commonwealth Fund, an organization that favors government-run health care and tailors its research conclusions to support that view. During the Senate debate over health reform, Sen. Kent Conrad (D-N.D.)

THE WORLD HEALTH SHAM RANKING SYSTEM

How is the U.S. ranked 37th in overall health performance, behind countries such as Oman, Morocco, Malta, and Andorra?

12.5% RESPONSIVENESS TO PATIENTS – The U.S. ranks No. 1 in this category.

25% HEALTH LEVEL – Disability adjusted life expectancy: affected by homicide rate, diet, tobacco use, etc.

25% HEALTH DISTRIBUTION – Variability of life expectancy: reflects behavior, incidence of violent crime in population subgroups, as well as disparities in medical care.

25% FINANCIAL FAIRNESS – Reflects the percentage of health care spending shouldered by the government.

12.5% RESPONSIVENESS DISTRIBUTION – Variability of health care experiences within a country.

The World Health Report 2000, World Health Organization

pointed to a large blue chart showing the United States in last place in health performance. "All of these countries have much lower costs than we do," he said, "and they have higher quality outcomes than ours."

Conrad was duped by a Commonwealth report published in *Health Affairs* in 2008 that puts the U.S. in 19th place due to diseases that are curable if treated soon enough.

Yet most of these deaths are caused by heart disease and circulatory diseases. The United States has a high incidence because for 50 years, Americans were the heaviest smokers and now are among the most obese. Bad behavior, not bad medicine, is to blame. Our health care system treats these diseases very effectively.

As the National Bureau of Economic Research concluded, "It seems inaccurate to attribute . . . high death rates from these causes to a poorly performing medical system."

Plus, while the Commonwealth researchers claimed to consider curable diseases of all sorts, they conspicuously omitted malignant prostate cancer – where U.S. care is stunningly successful. An American man diagnosed with it has a 99.3 percent chance of surviving it – far higher than in any Western European country. It's not a death sentence here, but in Scotland, only 71 percent survive, and in Germany, only 85 percent.

Conrad also trotted out another "pro-reform" statistic, pointing to a "shorter [U.S.] life expectancy compared with other industrialized countries." Again, demographers are quite clear on this: The causes of reduced U.S. life expectancy are our higher rates of auto fatalities and violent crime, plus half a century of excessive smoking – not bad medicine.

Setting the record straight, the National Bureau of Economic Research cautions that "the low longevity ranking of the United States is not likely to be a result of a poor functioning health care system."

The best measure of any nation's medical care is how likely *you* are to survive a serious illness and resume your previous active lifestyle. Cancer survival rates are unambiguous evidence of American achievement. Yet during the debate over health care reform, even National Breast Cancer Awareness Month was misused to promote the White House's agenda. If cancer runs in your family, this political propaganda could be dangerous to your health.

First Lady Michelle Obama stood with breast cancer survivors at a White House ceremony on Oct. 22, 2009, and claimed that American health care is "a system that only adds to the fear and stress that already comes with the disease."

The truth is, a woman diagnosed with breast cancer in the U.S. has a 90 percent chance of surviving it. In Europe, a woman's chance of survival is below 80 percent on average. These statistics, from the National Bureau of Economic Research, reflect the experiences of all women, not just those with insurance.

According to the bureau's research, women fare better in the U.S. because breast cancer is diagnosed earlier and treated more aggressively. Death rates from breast cancer have declined faster in the U.S. than anywhere else.

In the American system, there is a premium on the development of new detection methods and therapies. In other countries, government health programs delay adopting innovations in order to keep treatment costs down.

President Obama's Nobel Prize captured headlines in October 2009. But if breast cancer is a worry for you, three other Nobel Prizes awarded that month are more important. Scientists working in the U.S. took the Nobel Prize in Medicine for their research on how cancer cells continue to divide and duplicate far longer than healthy cells. Their research may hold the key to stopping the relentless growth of cancer.

Only one of these three Nobel scientists, Dr. Carol Greider, was born in the United States. The others were born in countries with government-run health care but chose to relocate to the U.S. to pursue their careers in medicine. Dr. Elizabeth Blackburn emigrated from Australia to the U.S. in the 1970s because, she told *The New York Times*, this country was "notably attractive" as a place to do research. Dr. Jack Szostak came from London.

The unrivaled pace of medical discovery in the U.S. is largely responsible for higher cancer survival rates here, according to the research bureau. Innovation is also responsible for about two-thirds of the annual increase in American health care spending, according to presidential adviser Blumenthal, writing in *The New England Journal of Medicine* in March 2001. Blumenthal and other advocates of ObamaCare want to slow down the adoption of new technologies. But no one battling cancer wants to settle for what oncologists had to offer a decade ago, and 10 years from now, no one will want to settle for 2010 treatments. The pace of innovation does add to costs, but it also gives families reason to hope.

Since 1950, the U.S. has won more Nobel Prizes in medicine and physiology than the rest of the world combined. If someone in your family is dealing with an illness still considered incurable, this is the nation of hope.

n *TheLancet.com* on Jan. 31, 2009, Dr.
anuel and co-authors presented a "com-
e lives system" for the allocation of very
ce resources, such as kidneys, vaccines,
ysis machines, and intensive care beds. Dr.
anuel makes a clear choice: "When imple-
ated, the complete lives system produces
iority curve on which individuals aged
ween roughly 15 and 40 years get the most
stantial chance, whereas the youngest and
est people get chances that are attenuated."
Dr. Emanuel concedes that his plan
ears to discriminate against older people,
he explains, "Unlike allocation by sex or
e, allocation by age is not invidious dis-
nination.... Treating 65-year-olds differ-
ly because of stereotypes or falsehoods
ald be ageist; treating them differently
ause they have already had more life-
rs is not."

The youngest are also put at the back of
line: "Adolescents have received substan-
education and parental care, investments
t will be wasted without a complete life.

Highest cancer survival rates and fastest
development of cures – compelling reasons
why this is the fight of our lifetime.

THE DANGEROUS IDEAS OF THE PRESIDENT'S MEDICAL ADVISER IN CHIEF

The new Obama health law puts important
decisions about your care in the hands of
presidential appointees. They will decide what
insurance plans cover, how much leeway your
doctor will have, and what seniors get under
Medicare. Chief among these advisers is Dr.
Ezekiel Emanuel, brother of White House
Chief of Staff Rahm Emanuel. Dr. Emanuel
has already been appointed to two key positions: health policy adviser at the Office of
Management and Budget and member of the
Federal Coordinating Council for Comparative Effectiveness Research.

Dr. Emanuel says that health care reform
will not be pain-free and that the usual recommendations for cutting medical spending
(often urged by the president) are mere

window dressing. As he wrote in the Feb. 27, 2008, issue of the *Journal of the American Medical Association*, or *JAMA*: "Vague promises of savings from cutting waste, enhancing prevention and wellness, installing electronic medical records, and improving quality are merely 'lipstick' cost control, more for show and public relations than for true change."

True reform, he argues, must include redefining doctors' ethical obligations. In the June 18, 2008, issue of *JAMA*, Dr. Emanuel blames the Hippocratic Oath for the "overuse" of medical care: "Medical school education and postgraduate education emphasize thoroughness," he writes. "This culture is further reinforced by a unique understanding of professional obligations, specifically the Hippocratic Oath's admonition to 'use my power to help the sick to the best of my ability and judgment' as an imperative to do everything for the patient regardless of cost or effect on others."

Dr. Emanuel chastises physicians for thinking only about their own patients' needs:

"Patients were to receive w
they needed, regardless of it
based on cost has been strenu
violated the Hippocratic Oat
with rationing, and derided a
on life."

"In the next decade, eve
face very hard choices abou
scarce medical resources," Er
in the Sept. 19, 2002, issue
land *Journal of Medicine*.

"You can't avoid these
Emanuel said in an Aug. 16,
in *The Washington Post*. "We h
versy in the United States wl
limited number of dialysis m
tle, they appointed what the
committee' to choose who sl
that committee was eventu
Society ended up paying th
dialysis instead of having pe
decisions." Emanuel obviou
comfortable than most of
notion of a panel or committ

En
ple
sca
dia
En
me
a
be
su
ol

ap
bu
ra
cri
en
wo
be
ye

th
tia
th

Highest cancer survival rates and fastest development of cures – compelling reasons why this is the fight of our lifetime.

THE DANGEROUS IDEAS OF THE PRESIDENT'S MEDICAL ADVISER IN CHIEF

The new Obama health law puts important decisions about your care in the hands of presidential appointees. They will decide what insurance plans cover, how much leeway your doctor will have, and what seniors get under Medicare. Chief among these advisers is Dr. Ezekiel Emanuel, brother of White House Chief of Staff Rahm Emanuel. Dr. Emanuel has already been appointed to two key positions: health policy adviser at the Office of Management and Budget and member of the Federal Coordinating Council for Comparative Effectiveness Research.

Dr. Emanuel says that health care reform will not be pain-free and that the usual recommendations for cutting medical spending (often urged by the president) are mere window dressing. As he wrote in the Feb. 27, 2008, issue of the *Journal of the American Medical Association*, or *JAMA*: "Vague promises of savings from cutting waste, enhancing prevention and wellness, installing electronic medical records, and improving quality are merely 'lipstick' cost control, more for show and public relations than for true change."

True reform, he argues, must include redefining doctors' ethical obligations. In the June 18, 2008, issue of *JAMA*, Dr. Emanuel blames the Hippocratic Oath for the "overuse" of medical care: "Medical school education and postgraduate education emphasize thoroughness," he writes. "This culture is further reinforced by a unique understanding of professional obligations, specifically the Hippocratic Oath's admonition to 'use my power to help the sick to the best of my ability and judgment' as an imperative to do everything for the patient regardless of cost or effect on others."

Dr. Emanuel chastises physicians for thinking only about their own patients' needs:

"Patients were to receive whatever services they needed, regardless of its cost. Reasoning based on cost has been strenuously resisted; it violated the Hippocratic Oath, was associated with rationing, and derided as putting a price on life."

"In the next decade, every country will face very hard choices about how to allocate scarce medical resources," Emanuel predicted in the Sept. 19, 2002, issue of *The New England Journal of Medicine.*

"You can't avoid these questions," Dr. Emanuel said in an Aug. 16, 2009, interview in *The Washington Post.* "We had a big controversy in the United States when there were a limited number of dialysis machines. In Seattle, they appointed what they called a 'God committee' to choose who should get it, and that committee was eventually abandoned. Society ended up paying the whole bill for dialysis instead of having people make those decisions." Emanuel obviously feels more comfortable than most of us do with the notion of a panel or committee playing God.

In *TheLancet.com* on Jan. 31, 2009, Dr. Emanuel and co-authors presented a "complete lives system" for the allocation of very scarce resources, such as kidneys, vaccines, dialysis machines, and intensive care beds. Dr. Emanuel makes a clear choice: "When implemented, the complete lives system produces a priority curve on which individuals aged between roughly 15 and 40 years get the most substantial chance, whereas the youngest and oldest people get chances that are attenuated."

Dr. Emanuel concedes that his plan appears to discriminate against older people, but he explains, "Unlike allocation by sex or race, allocation by age is not invidious discrimination. . . . Treating 65-year-olds differently because of stereotypes or falsehoods would be ageist; treating them differently because they have already had more life-years is not."

The youngest are also put at the back of the line: "Adolescents have received substantial education and parental care, investments that will be wasted without a complete life.

Infants, by contrast, have not yet received these investments."

Dr. Emanuel urged the president to push forward with the Obama health law, no matter how intensely Americans opposed it. On Nov. 16, 2008, he recommended that the president use Chicago-style arm-twisting if necessary. "If the automakers want a bailout, then they and their suppliers have to agree to support and lobby for the administration's health care reform effort."

That's how the Obama health law got passed.

MEDICARE'S PROPOSED RATIONER IN CHIEF DONALD BERWICK

On April 19, 2010, President Obama nominated Dr. Donald Berwick to head the Centers for Medicare & Medicaid Services. Berwick is a dangerous choice for seniors and baby boomers who will be depending on Medicare.

Berwick confesses to having a love affair – a "romance," he says – with the British National Health Service. In a speech commemorating the NHS's 60th anniversary, he praises its orderliness, frugality, redistribution of wealth, and explicit rationing. "Behold the mess – the far bigger, costlier, unfair mess" that is health care in the U.S., he says.

Berwick has radical plans to transform American medical care. He laid them out in his "Triple Aim" plan published in 2008 in *Health Affairs*. He concedes the "pain of the transition" will entail "the disruption of institutions, forms, habits, beliefs, and income streams in the status quo...." The new Obama health law will allow Berwick to transform Medicare without any further approval by Congress or the American public. The law authorizes the executive branch to create pilot programs – reorganizing how and where patients are treated, what choices they have, how their doctors are paid, and what medical services they can get – and then expand these programs on a nationwide basis as quickly as possible.

When the president campaigned for his health legislation, he told people with insurance not to worry. If you like your doctor and your coverage, you won't have to change, he repeatedly promised. Americans didn't vote for the pain of transition. Yet Berwick's writings indicate the large changes in store for Medicare patients.

First, expect an environment of medical scarcity, meaning fewer MRIs and other equipment and longer waits to be treated. Applauding the British system at its anniversary, he said, "You [the NHS] plan the supply; you aim a bit low; historically, you prefer slightly too little of a technology or service to much too much; and then you search for care bottlenecks and try to relieve them."

Second, expect that your own health choices will be "managed" by a "medical home." You will no longer be the one deciding when to see a doctor or consult a specialist. Medical home is this decade's version of HMO-style medicine, according to the Congressional Budget Office, with a primary care provider to oversee your access to costly services such as visits to specialists and diagnostic tests. In his "Triple Aim" plan, Berwick says not to expect your primary care provider to be a physician. Many, perhaps most, will be nurses or physician's assistants. Currently, Medicare patients can decide to see a doctor and Medicare pays. Not in the future.

Worse still, if you do get to a doctor, don't expect the doctor to be able to make decisions based on your individual case. Physician autonomy is a thing of the past, argues Berwick, who wrote an essay called "The Epitaph of Profession" in the 2009 *British Journal of General Practice*.

Berwick earned accolades for his 100,000 Lives Campaign, a superb effort to codify and disseminate guidelines to keep patients safe from infections, bedsores, and other unintended consequences of medical care. In the area of patient safety, guidelines should be rigorously enforced. There are no disagreements about the need for clean hands. Patient safety rules are like the rules a pilot follows in the cockpit. But beyond patient safety, in fields from cardiology to obstetrics, there are numerous disagreements on what are best practices. Yet Berwick argues aggressively for almost eliminating physician leeway.

In his "Triple Aim" plan, Berwick deplores the American heath care system as "designed to respond to the acute needs of individual patients." His plan is to "anticipate and shape patterns of care for important subgroups." Subgroups could be defined by age, affliction, or socioeconomic status. Woe to you if you're not in a favored subgroup or part of the plan. In his beloved British National Health Service, those decisions are made by what he lauds as the "maddening, majestic machinery of politics." The elderly fare poorly in that system, as you can see by visiting a ward reserved for their care in a British hospital. You will find long rows of beds, sometimes even without a privacy curtain, and cancer survival rates far lower than current survival rates in the U.S.

* * *

Second Opinions from America's Leading Physicians

Many physicians understood the dire consequences of the Obama proposals for their own patients. President Obama didn't consult with them. But on Oct. 19, 2009, a group of highly regarded physicians assembled at the Grand Hyatt hotel in New York City. Here is what they had to say on the fundamental issues:

On Treating the Elderly

Dr. Seymour Cohen, oncologist, named to "America's Top Doctors": "When we went to medical school, people used to die at 66, 67 and 68. Medicare paid for two or three years. Social Security paid for two or three years. We're the bad guys. We're responsible for keeping people alive to 85. So we're now going to try to change health care because people are living too long. It just doesn't make very good sense to me."

Shifting Resources From Specialty to Primary Care

Dr. Jeffrey Moses, interventional cardiologist, named to "America's Top Doctors": "If you have heart failure or heart attack or coronaries in general in the hospital you need to be treated by a cardiologist. Study after study shows that ... when you have an illness and you want to have an accurate diagnosis and the most up-to-date and accurate treatment, you want a specialist."

Patient Privacy

Dr. Samuel Guillory, ophthalmologist, refractive and orbital surgery, named to Castle Connolly's "New York's Top Doctors": "We're being asked by the executive branch ... to break the code with patients and deliver all their records into electronic medical records. ..."

Cost-Cutting Methods

Dr. David Fields, obstetrician and gynecologist, Lenox Hill Hospital, New York: "Government is in the process of duplicating everything that managed care did for the last 15 years that was reviled by everybody and which we fought very hard to overcome.... Capitation was the worst thing that ever happened to medical care."

Dr. Tracy Pfeifer, plastic surgeon, former president, New York Regional Society of Plastic Surgeons: "When physicians graduate from medical school we take an oath, the Hippocratic Oath, to do no harm to our patients.... These government programs that are being proposed I think are very scary in the sense that physicians could be induced to violate the Hippocratic Oath."

Dr. Joel Kassimir, dermatologist, Mount Sinai Hospital, New York: "We're now being told by physicians advising the president that we take the Hippocratic Oath too seriously."

A 20-Page Bill in Plain English to Reduce Premiums and Help Laid-Off Americans

This Bill Is Not Dangerous to Your Health or Your Freedom

Contains No Mandates Forcing Individuals or States to Do Anything

Every day, Americans tell me they want a bill written in plain English. They want members of Congress to read the entire bill before voting. They want a bill anyone can inspect. A 20-page bill means that pork projects, secret deals, and exemptions for Washington insiders cannot be slipped between the pages. The language in this bill does not give the American people the runaround.

Twenty pages should be enough. The framers of the Constitution established the entire federal government in just 18 pages.

This bill recognizes that states have regulated health insurance for more than six decades, consistent with the McCarran-Ferguson Act of 1945. Some states have taken smart approaches to lowering costs and expanding access, especially to people with pre-existing conditions. This bill copies what works.

TITLE 1: Liberates consumers to buy policies from other states and puts consumers on notice that the products they buy out-of-state may have different consumer protections than those imposed in their own state. This title also imposes federal consumer protections on plans sold interstate, ensuring that those plans prohibit rescission and protect consumers who have paid their premiums from being dropped. An HMO plan costs a 25-year-old California male $260 a month, while a New Yorker has to pay $1,228 for a similar plan. Free the New Yorker to shop outside of his state.

TITLE 2: Provides federal incentives for states to establish medical courts, ensuring quicker, fairer verdicts in medical liability cases and at the same time preserving every litigant's right to trial by jury. Medical courts will be presided over by a judge who knows the issues, has the experience, and can identify honest expert witnesses. (The judge will also reduce the impact of those who are not honest. Tort law has always been a matter left to states.) This bill does not mandate that states establish medical courts or attempt to federalize tort law. It does provide block grants to states to impose caps on damages and, more importantly, to establish medical courts. Why just cap unjust damage awards when you can eliminate them by having expert judges?

TITLE 3: Provides federal incentives for states to establish or improve subsidized high-risk pools to help consumers with preexisting conditions and poor health. (This concept is similar to what is also proposed in the Patients' Choice Act, supported by Sen. Tom Coburn (R-Okla.). No state is required to establish these pools.)

TITLE 4: Extends the current 65 percent COBRA subsidy, established by the American Recovery and Reinvestment Act of 2009. The president's fiscal year 2011 budget also contains such an extension. Republicans are likely to find this an important common ground. COBRA subsidies are not a permanent entitlement but rather a temporary helping hand to those who have been laid off. The average COBRA annual premium for a family of four is $13,322, a big price tag when you've lost your job. For more than half of uninsured Americans legally in this country, being uninsured is a temporary problem. They find another job and are insured again in less than a year. We need to help them in between jobs. The 10-year cost of Titles 1, 2, and 3 of this bill is $27 billion. The COBRA extension is already included in the president's fiscal year 2011 budget. Funding this COBRA subsidy could cost $24 billion per year and provide coverage for an estimated 7 million people.

You can read the entire bill at: www.defendyourhealthcare.us.

When you're told that "something had to be done" and the "Obama health law is better than nothing," you have the answer: Here is a 20-page bill that will help make insurance affordable and help the uninsured. It can be done without lowering your standard of care, putting the government in charge of your care, or taking away your freedom.

The American people should be calling on the president and Congress to repeal the ObamaCare law.

First American edition published in 2010 by Encounter Books,
an activity of Encounter for Culture and Education, Inc.,
a nonprofit, tax exempt corporation.
Encounter Books website address: www.encounterbooks.com

Manufactured in the United States and printed on
acid-free paper. The paper used in this publication meets
the minimum requirements of ANSI/NISO Z39.48–1992
(R 1997) (*Permanence of Paper*).

FIRST AMERICAN EDITION

LIBRARY OF CONGRESS CATALOGING-IN-PUBLICATION DATA

Ross, Betsy McCaughey, 1948–
Obama health law : what it says and how to overturn it / Betsy
McCaughey.
p.   cm. — (Encounter broadsides)
ISBN-13: 978-1-59403-506-7 (pbk. : alk. paper)
ISBN-10: 1-59403-506-7 (pbk. : alk. paper)
1. United States. Patient Protection and Affordable Care Act—Popu-
lar works. 2. Health insurance—Law and legislation—United
States—Popular works. 3. National health insurance—Law and leg-
islation—United States—Popular works. 4. Health care reform—
United States—Popular works. I. Title.
KF3605.A328201A2   2010
344.7302'2—dc22
2010019357

10 9 8 7 6 5 4 3 2 1